"From revised vegan versions of peanut butter cups, Laura gets us up to date with nostalgic classics one easy recipe after another in *The Little Vegan Dessert Cookbook*. Full of fun photos and graphics, it's a page turner! My absolute favorites are the luscious gluten free bourbon balls and creamy chocolate mints, both of which are refreshingly decadent and uncomplicated."

— *Dustin Harder, Chef, Author, Television Host, and Creator of The Vegan Roadie*

"I'm glad that Laura has taken the time to reflect on these historical tomes. There is no harm in loving a recipe and putting your own touch on it. Substituting regional products or adjusting for dietary needs simply adds personality to your table . . . go for it. The stories that you recreate are now yours, but don't forget the roots in your favorite old cookbook."

— *Tom Douglas, Celebrity Chef and James Beard Award Winner*

"For over three decades, Laura has been baking healthy desserts using vegan ingredients. Her treats are scooped up as soon as they hit the dessert counter at my restaurant because they're delicious, healthy and guilt-free. Treat yourself to this book and explore the world of vegan baking. You'll be happy that you did!"

— *Stephan Germano, CEO of the Pasta Pizza Store, former head chef of the award-winning eatery, the New York Pizza Factory*

"I have had the honor of being the lucky recipient of Laura's bourbon balls for many years while she diligently and thoughtfully developed this book, and they do not disappoint! These delightful treats are just one of the many winning, modernized recipes in Laura's heart-warming ode to your grandparent's kitchen."

— *Cortney Anderson-Sanford, NBC TV-winning cook, Lifestylist and Etiquette Revolutionary*

"Laura's book—filled with mouthwatering recipes for delicious cookies, cakes, and confections—goes a step further towards enabling us to enjoy the fun of making them whilst feeling comfortable that we can avoid the daily food-stuff unnecessarily loaded with animal products.

"It's a treat to know that vegans can continue to enjoy scrumptious desserts while maintaining the healthy positive effects of vegan food on BMI, cholesterol and, combined with other healthy lifestyle choices, reducing the risk of cancer."

— *Dr. Ardiana Beeley MD, PhD, Specialist in Public Health Medicine, London, England*

"Cookbooks are definitely a passion for Laura. She has spent so much time and energy collecting and studying old cookbooks... We all have cravings for sweets and Laura's recipes certainly satisfy those cravings in a delicious and very healthy way! [Her] attention to detail will make *The Little Vegan Dessert Cookbook* a favorite in your home. Her desserts not only look great, they taste great. . . . Please enjoy Laura's recipes. I hope that they will become traditions for you."

— *Barbara Nicklaus, author of the cookbook,* Well Done! *and wife of world-renowned golf legend Jack Nicklaus*

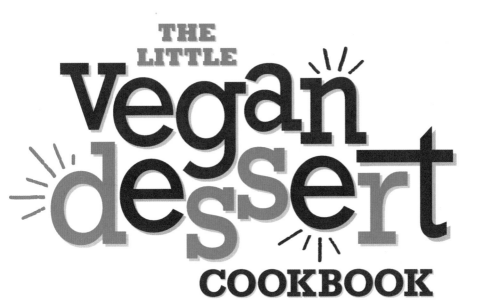

THE LITTLE Vegan dessert COOKBOOK

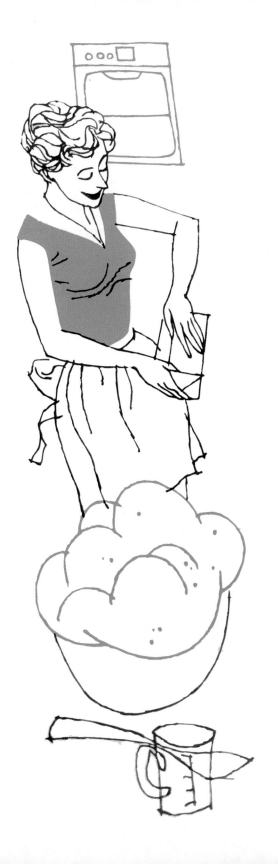

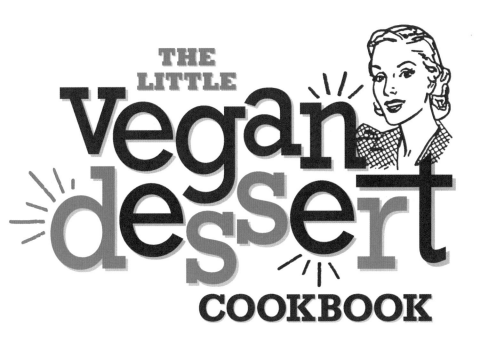

THE LITTLE vegan dessert COOKBOOK

VINTAGE RECIPES REVISED

by Laura Crotty

Lincoln Square Books
New York, NY

Cover design by Gus Yoo
Book interior design by Kerry Tinger
Author photo by Gretchen Taylor

ISBN: 978-1-947187-11-5

Library of Congress Control Number: 2020933792

Lincoln Square Books
New York, NY
www.lincolnsquarebooks.com

ACKNOWLEDGMENTS

I would like to thank some wonderfully
talented people who helped facilitate the
publication of this book. Thanks to Peter Rubie
for his belief in my work and ever-present
guidance. I would also like to thank
Tom Douglas for his generosity and support,
Dave Makin for standing behind this project,
and Paul Cohen and Kerry Tinger.
I am forever grateful for your combined
expertise and insight.

"Life is uncertain. Eat dessert first."

– *Ernestine Ulmer*

Table of Contents

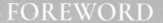

FOREWORD

BY TOM DOUGLAS

What is it about old cookbooks? They keep the fires burning for a time and place. They breathe like a red-hot wok just hit with a fresh Dungeness crab or velvety soy-marinated pork loin. When you crack the cover of one, it feels like a research project in a pre-internet encyclopedia, and yet the recipes come to life, quickly enveloping your senses with memories of birthday celebrations, first dinner dates, and tragic recipes gone awry.

I learned to cook alongside many talented chefs and gleaned from others whose words and techniques imbedded in cookbooks were my only guide. Our popular cookbook dinner series in 1984 at the acclaimed Café Sport in Seattle was a revelation in cooking styles, attitudes, and most importantly, a commitment to a recipe from beginning to end. Some books are light on recipes and preachy on theory like the *Chez Panisse Menu Cookbook*, my all-time favorite. Others are eye-popping, palette-changing monsters that influence the rest of your cooking career, like Barbara Tropps' *The Modern Art of Chinese Cooking*.

The vintage cookbooks I acquire today have a few things in common. I love books with handwritten comments, ruminations about the cook's efforts for the recipe, whether it worked the way the author designed it or eventually how their guest enjoyed the final product. I treasure signed first editions in fine shape. Really though, any cookbook, old or new inspires me to get off my butt, get in the kitchen, and enjoy a trip through someone else's idea of a terrific plum of a recipe!

I'm glad that Laura is taking the time to reflect on these historical tomes. There is no harm in loving a recipe and putting your own touch on it. Substituting regional products or adjusting for dietary needs simply adds personality to your table. Cooking techniques change over time like fashion and taste buds...go for it. The stories that you recreate are now yours, but don't forget the roots in your favorite old cookbook.

Tom Douglas is an executive chef, author, radio talk show host and restaurateur known for winning the James Beard Award multiple times, including distinctions for Best Northwest Chef, Best Restaurateur and Best American Cookbook.

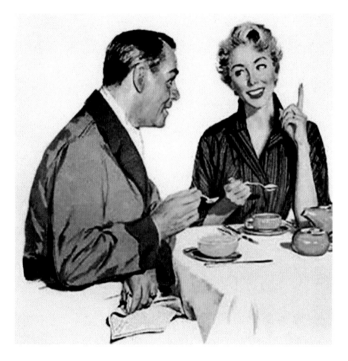

The idea for this cookbook hatched years ago after launching *Broiled Grapefruit* (now @ lauracrotty.com), a blog founded to showcase revised, vintage recipes. Tired of paying retail prices for commercially produced plant-based treats, I developed these recipes out of necessity. The desserts presented are not only cost efficient but deliciously satisfying. Inside you will find classic dessert recipes that were adapted for those interested in plant-based eating. While retaining the history and stylistic elements of certain decades in time, these recipes were inspired by my cherished and ever-expanding collection of old cookbooks. Although the collection spans centuries, I gravitate towards books from the 1950s, 60s, and 70s because of the ingredients that were used, as well as certain design features.

I hope this cookbook earns a well-worn place on your shelf and inspires you to dig up some old recipes of your own. After all, old recipes aren't just words on a page, they are the tastes, flavors, and textures that bring us back to a certain place in time, and we all have our favorites. Good luck and happy baking!

– *Laura Crotty*

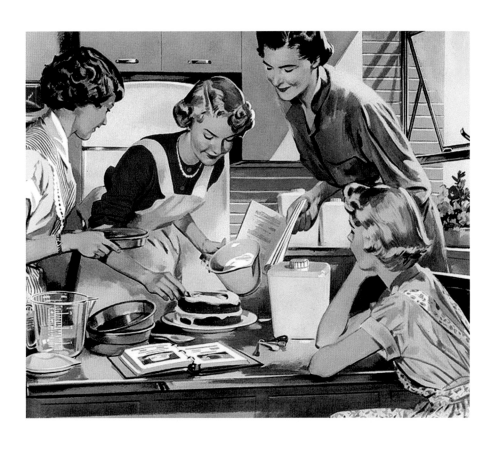

PANTRY ITEMS

Some of the ingredients used in this cookbook may be unfamiliar to you. However, don't be surprised if you find yourself using them as substitutes in your own recipes. All of these ingredients are readily available at most grocery stores, so there will be no need to pay the inflated prices charged at many health food chains.

GROUND FLAXSEED
Derived from flax (also called linseed), one of the oldest crops in the world, flaxseed is known to have been cultivated in ancient China and Egypt. Flaxseed is a source of fiber, antioxidants, and healthy fat.

QUINOA FLOUR
Quinoa flour comes from a plant in the goosefoot family. Even though we think of it as a grain, it is actually the seeds of the quinoa plant. Quinoa is also a complete protein containing all of the nine essential amino acids and is gluten free as well. There are hundreds of varieties but white, red, and black are the most commonly cultivated.

SPELT FLOUR
Spelt flour comes from the ancient grain spelt or hulled wheat and is a primitive relative to modern-day wheat. Although it is a member of the same grain family, it is an entirely different species. Spelt has been cultivated since 5000 BC and has a mellower, nuttier flavor than traditional wheat flour.

OAT MILK

Oat milk is made by soaking whole-grain oats
in water, blending them and then straining
the mixture. It is a smooth-tasting, non-dairy
substitute that I use often in baking. It is available
in most stores in a variety of flavors, but I used
plain for these recipes.

COCONUT SUGAR

Produced from the sap of flower buds from the
coconut palm, it is not to be confused with palm
sugar which is from a different type of palm tree.
Coconut sugar is a mild alternative to processed
sugar and because it is unrefined, it retains all of
its natural vitamins and minerals. It has a deep
caramel color and is slightly sweet.

AQUAFABA

Aquafaba is the name used for the cooking liquid
of beans and other legumes like chickpeas. It is the
liquid found in canned beans from the store, or the
liquid that remains after you cook your own beans.
I use canned Great Northern bean liquid for these
recipes, but any bean liquid will do. If the bean
liquid is too watery, reduce it in a saucepan until
its consistency thickens and resembles that of an
egg white.

BAKING TIPS

Here are a few tips that may come in handy when using the recipes in this cookbook.

SUBSTITUTIONS
If you don't have the exact ingredients, experiment.

Get to know the ingredients well before substituting. A little bit of research on a particular ingredient will prevent mistakes along the way when baking.

EGG REPLACEMENT
Try different methods

1 egg equals:

- 1/4 cup mashed banana (keep in mind that your recipe will have a hint of banana flavor)

- 1 teaspoon of no-taste vegetable oil, plus 2 teaspoons baking powder, plus 2 tablespoons of water

- 1 tablespoon ground flaxseed plus 3 tablespoons of water (let sit until thickened, about 5 minutes)

CHOCOLATE

For non-dairy semi-sweet chocolate, I used Baker's brand semi-sweet chocolate bars.

SALT

I use fine-grain sea salt for these recipes, but if you don't have it on hand, regular iodized salt works as well. Just make sure it is not a course grain.

NON-DAIRY BUTTER

I use Earth Balance soy-free, non-dairy, tub-spread for butter in these recipes, but other Earth Balance varieties work just as well. Smart Balance brand is also a great choice.

VEGAN BATTERS

It is important to know that vegan batters tend to be thicker than traditional egg batters; at times they can resemble the consistency of frosting, as is the case with my chocolate brownie recipe. Just scoop out the batter into the prepared pan and bake accordingly.

8

COOKIES

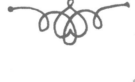

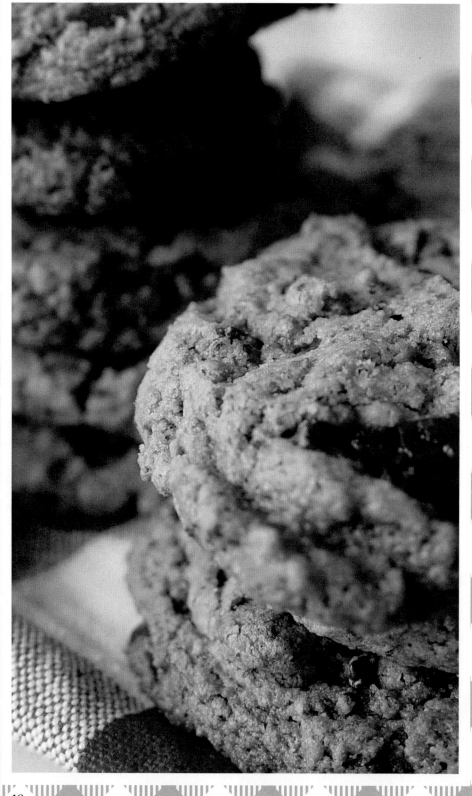

chocolate chip

I revised this 1937 Toll House Inn classic. Luckily for us, Ruth Wakefield's attempt at a chocolate butter cookie failed and the chocolate chip was born.

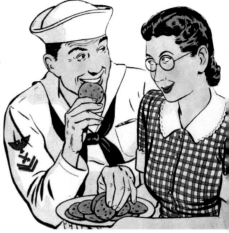

yield: 2 dozen cookies

2 cups oat flour

1/2 teaspoon baking soda

1/2 teaspoon salt

1/3 cup non-dairy butter

1/3 cup non-hydrogenated vegetable shortening

1 cup coconut sugar

3 tablespoon water

1 tablespoon ground flaxseeds

1 teaspoon vanilla

8 ounces non-dairy semi-sweet chocolate bar roughly chopped into about 1/2-inch pieces

1. Preheat the oven to 350 degrees.

2. In a small bowl, sift together the flour, baking soda, and salt.

3. Mix the ground flax seeds and water together in another bowl.

4. In a larger bowl, cream together the butter, shortening, sugar, and vanilla.

5. Add the flaxseed mixture to the large bowl and after incorporated, gradually add the dry ingredients, mixing well with each addition.

6. Fold in the chocolate and drop by rounded tablespoons onto ungreased cookie sheets.

7. Bake for 8 to 10 minutes.

rustic linzer tarts

Inspired by Luchow's Linzer Torte from Luchow's 1952 German Cookbook, I developed this recipe when I was in culinary school. They're wonderfully wholesome.

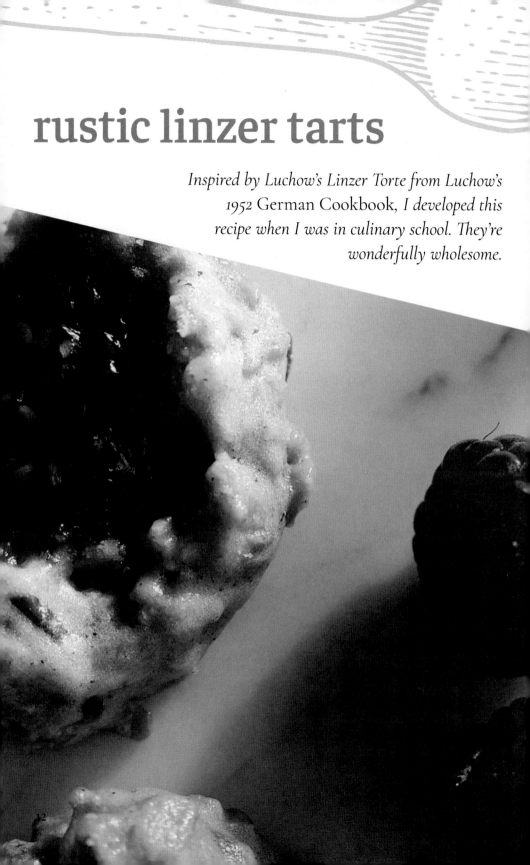

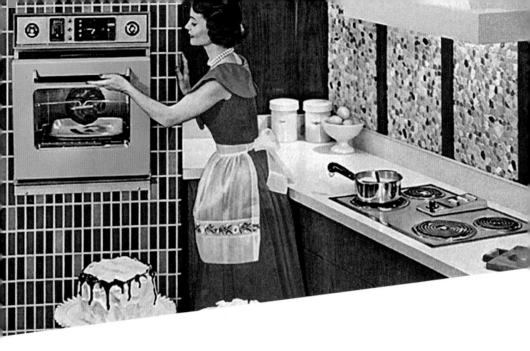

yield: about 2 dozen cookies

1 cup finely chopped pecans

1 cup rolled oats

1 cup of all-purpose flour

Pinch of sea salt

1/4 teaspoon cinnamon

1/2 cup corn oil

1/2 cup maple syrup

1/4-1/2 cup raspberry jam

1. Preheat the oven to 350 degrees.

2. In a large bowl, mix the oats, flour, salt, and cinnamon together.

3. In a smaller bowl, combine the corn oil and maple syrup.

4. Add the corn oil mixture to the dry ingredients until combined. Stir in the pecans.

5. Drop by rounded tablespoons onto ungreased cookie sheets. Press the top of each cookie with the pad of thumb to form an indent. Place 1 teaspoon of the raspberry jam inside the indent and repeat with each cookie.

6. Bake for 8 to 10 minutes or until edges begin to brown.

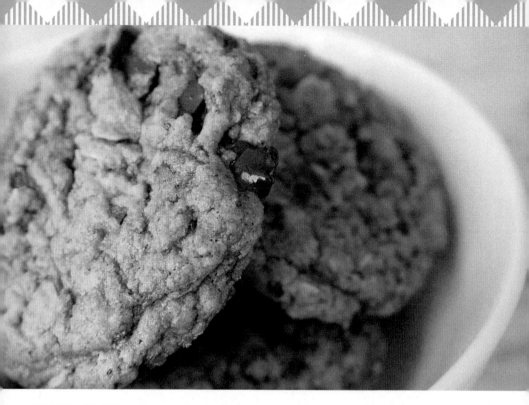

When I was on break during my second year in college, I used to drive over the George Washington Bridge from our home in New Jersey to purchase a particular vegan peanut butter cookie from a small deli in downtown Manhattan. In 1989, this single, wrapped cookie, sweetened only with barley malt, was about $2.79.

Even back then, health foods were pricey, and sweet treats were just as expensive, but that didn't stop me from seeking out this very special cookie. My interest in baking non-dairy desserts led me to culinary school after college, where I learned how to make vegan treats at home. This peanut butter cookie was one of the first recipes that I developed. I used to sell it at my brother's restaurant to all of the moms seeking healthier, non-processed desserts for their kids. Now you can bake these cookies at home and enjoy not only saving money, but providing wholesome desserts for your loved ones.

14

peanut butter cookies

This recipe features the winning combination of creamy peanut butter and rich dark chocolate chunks. Revised from the Favorite Desserts of America Cookbook, *dated 1968.*

yield: about 30 cookies

2 ³/₄ cups all-purpose flour

1 ¹/₂ cups rolled oats

1/2 tablespoon baking powder

1/2 tablespoon salt

1/2 cup creamy peanut butter

1 cup corn oil

1 ¹/₂ cups coconut sugar

1 ¹/₂ cups maple syrup

1 tablespoon vanilla

3 tablespoons water

1 tablespoon ground flaxseed

2 cups non-dairy semi-sweet baking chocolate chopped into 1/2-inch pieces

1. Preheat the oven to 350 degrees.

2. In a medium bowl, mix the flour, oats, baking powder, and salt together.

3. Mix the ground flaxseeds and water together in a small bowl and set aside to thicken, about 5 minutes.

4. In a larger bowl, combine the peanut butter, corn oil, coconut sugar, maple syrup, and vanilla. Stir in the flaxseed mixture.

5. Add the dry ingredients to the wet gradually, mixing well with each addition. Fold in the chopped chocolate.

6. Drop by rounded tablespoons onto ungreased cookie sheets and bake for 8 to 15 minutes.

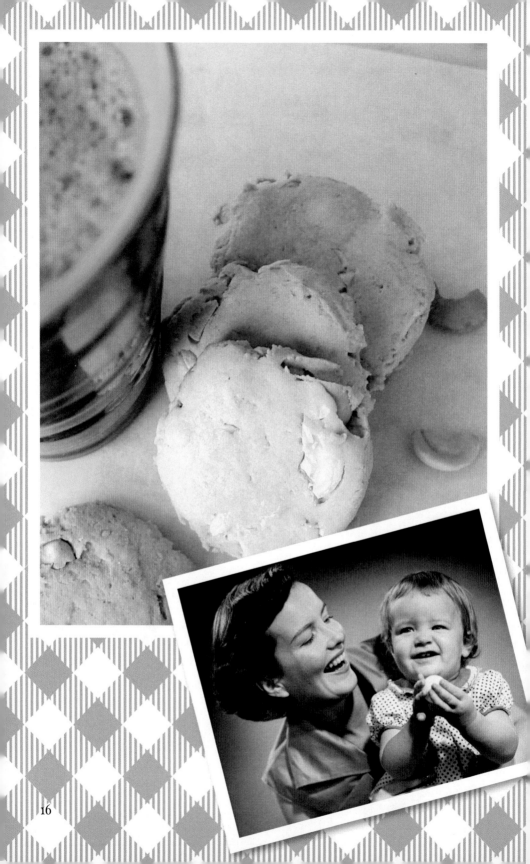

sand tarts

The cashews add a creamy richness to this cookie, which is similar to the classic Pecan Sandie; revised from The American Everyday Cookbook sand tart recipe, dated 1955.

yield: 2 dozen cookies

2 cups all-purpose flour

1 1/4 cups cashews, chopped

1/2 cup corn oil

1/4 cup non-dairy butter

3/4 cup maple syrup

1/4 teaspoon salt

1. Preheat the oven to 350 degrees.

2. In a medium bowl, mix the flour, salt, and cashews.

3. In a separate larger bowl, cream the non-dairy butter, add the maple syrup and corn oil, and mix well.

4. Gradually add the flour mixture and mix thoroughly.

5. Drop by rounded tablespoons onto ungreased cookie sheets. The batter will be a little crumbly. Press the batter together when placing the spoonfuls on the baking sheet, and lightly flatten with the heel of your hand.

6. Bake for about 8 to 10 minutes or until edges start to brown. Remove from cookie sheet to cool.

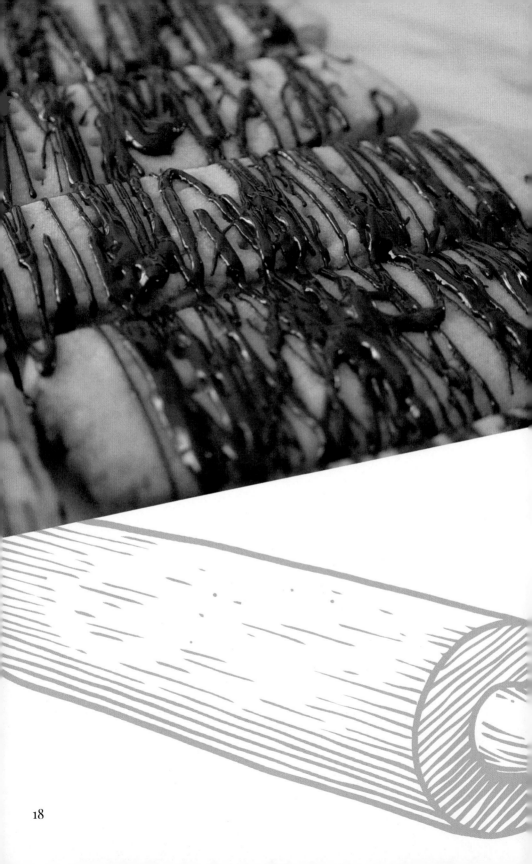

shortbread

This decadent cookie is incredibly satisfying and easy to make; revised from Amy Vanderbilt's Complete Cookbook for Scotch Shortbread, *dated 1961.*

yield: 5 dozen cookies

2 cups non-dairy butter at room temperature

1 cup coconut sugar

4 ½ cups all-purpose flour

4 ounces of semi-sweet non-dairy baking chocolate, chopped

1. Preheat the oven to 325 degrees.

2. In a large bowl, cream the non-dairy butter and coconut sugar together. Gradually add 3 to 3 3/4 cups flour. Mix well until the dough starts to come together.

3. Sprinkle work surface with the remaining flour. Knead the dough for five minutes, adding enough flour to make a soft dough.

4. Roll out dough to 1/2-inch in thickness. Cut the dough into 3x1-inch strips and place onto ungreased baking sheets.

5. Pierce the strips horizontally with a fork and bake for 20 to 25 minutes. Remove onto racks to cool.

6. In a microwave-proof bowl, place the semi-sweet chocolate. Heat in 30-second intervals, stirring in between, until thoroughly melted and smooth.

7. Drizzle the melted chocolate with a spoon over the shortbread and leave to cool completely.

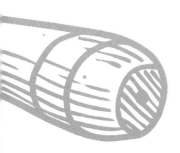

oatmeal cookies

I love potato chips and adding them to this Oatmeal Raisin Cookie was just magic. Revised from the Farm Journal's Country Cookbook, *dated 1959.*

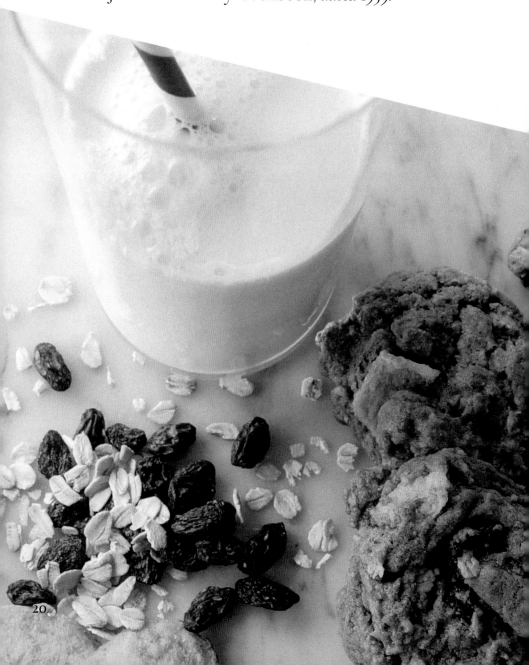

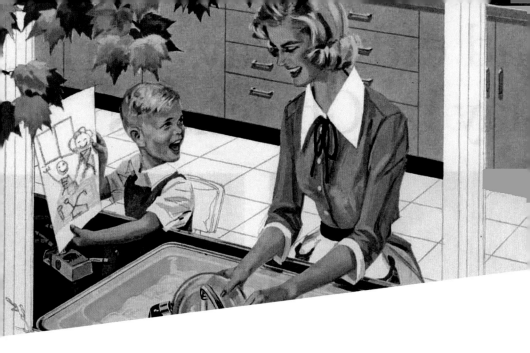

yield: about 3 dozen cookies

1 cup non-dairy butter at room temperature

1 ³/₄ cups coconut sugar

6 tablespoons aquafaba

1 ¹/₂ teaspoons vanilla extract

1 ¹/₂ teaspoons baking soda

2 ¹/₂ cups spelt flour

1 cup rolled oats

1 cup raisins

1 ¹/₂ cups potato chips

1. Preheat the oven to 325 degrees. Grease cookie sheets.

2. In a medium bowl cream the non-dairy butter and coconut sugar together. Mix in the bean liquid and vanilla extract.

3. In a larger bowl, combine the baking soda, spelt flour, and oats.

4. Add the creamed mixture to the flour and mix well. Fold in the raisins and potato chips.

5. Drop by rounded tablespoons onto cookie sheets and bake for 10 minutes. Oven times may vary, so keep an eye on these and remove from the oven when the edges start to brown.

genets

I still have the index card that my grandmother gave to me with her original recipe for this light Italian lemon cookie. It dates back to the early 1940s.

yield: 18 two-inch cookies

for the cookies:

1/4 cup water

1 tablespoon non-hydrogenated vegetable shortening

1/4 cup of non-dairy butter at room temperature

1/2 cup sugar

1 tablespoon plus 4 teaspoons baking powder, separated

1 1/2 plus 1/4 cups all-purpose flour, separated

2 tablespoons lemon extract

for the icing:

1 cup confectioners sugar

1-2 tablespoons lemon extract

1. Preheat the oven to 350 degrees.

2. In a small bowl mix the water, shortening, 1/4 cup flour, and 2 teaspoons of baking powder; set aside.

3. In a separate large bowl, cream the non-dairy butter, sugar, and lemon extract together; add the vegetable oil mixture and mix well.

4. In a medium bowl, mix the flour and remaining baking powder. Gradually add the dry ingredients to the butter mixture, mixing well with your hands or a spoon. Continue to add more flour until the dough is no longer sticky and starts to come together. Knead lightly, being careful not to overwork the dough. You want it to be soft or the cookies will be tough.

5. Drop by rounded tablespoons onto ungreased cookie sheets two inches apart; bake for 10 to 12 minutes. Let cool on rack and drizzle with icing.

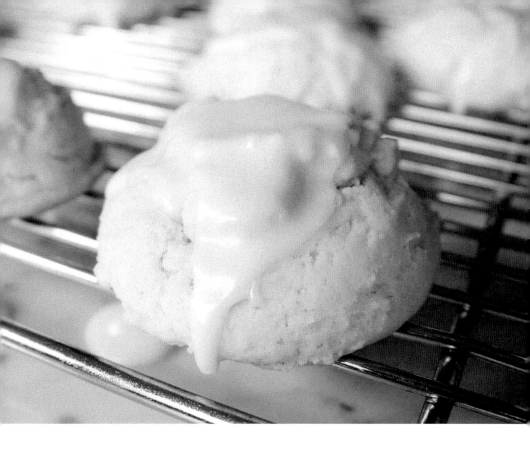

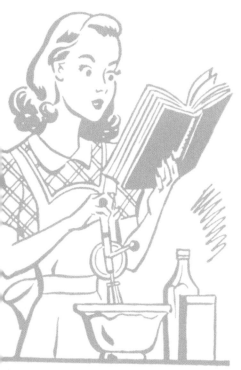

directions for the icing:

1. Mix 1 cup of confectioners sugar with the lemon extract until it starts to come together.

2. Add 1-2 teaspoons of water at a time until the icing is loose enough to drizzle. Go slow, you don't want to dilute the icing too much.

3. With a teaspoon, drizzle the icing over the cookies while on the rack. Cool completely and store in an airtight container.

24

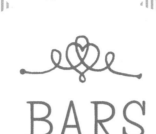

BARS

chocolate pie bars

I turned this 1962 American Woman's Cookbook *recipe for chocolate pie into rich ganache bars and switched out the store-bought pastry with a homemade graham cracker crust.*

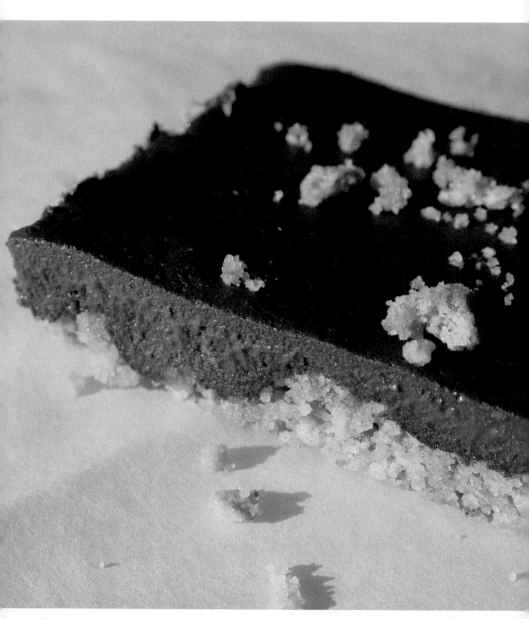

yield: 12 *squares*

for the crust:

1 ½ cups graham cracker crumbs (extra for topping)

1/4 cup confectioners sugar

6 tablespoons non-dairy butter, melted

for the pie:

1 cup non-dairy vanilla creamer

8 ounces of non-dairy semi-sweet chocolate, chopped

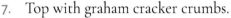

1. Preheat the oven to 375 degrees.

2. In a small bowl, mix the graham crumbs, sugar, and non-dairy butter together until crumbly.

3. Press into an 8x8-inch square pan and bake for 10 minutes; set aside.

4. In a microwave-safe bowl, add the chopped chocolate and non-dairy creamer. Heat in 30-second intervals until melted.

5. Stir mixture until smooth and pour into crust.

6. Refrigerate for 4 hours or until set.

7. Top with graham cracker crumbs.

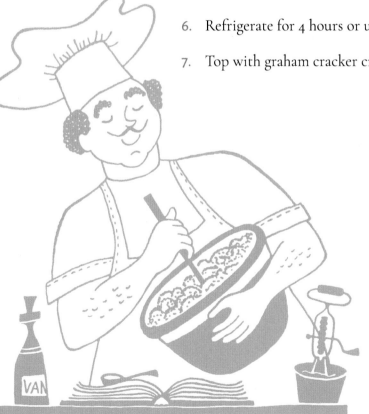

brownies

I cut out the shortening and eggs from this 1961 Betty Crocker Picture Cookbook recipe. No one will know that these rich and decadent brownies are vegan.

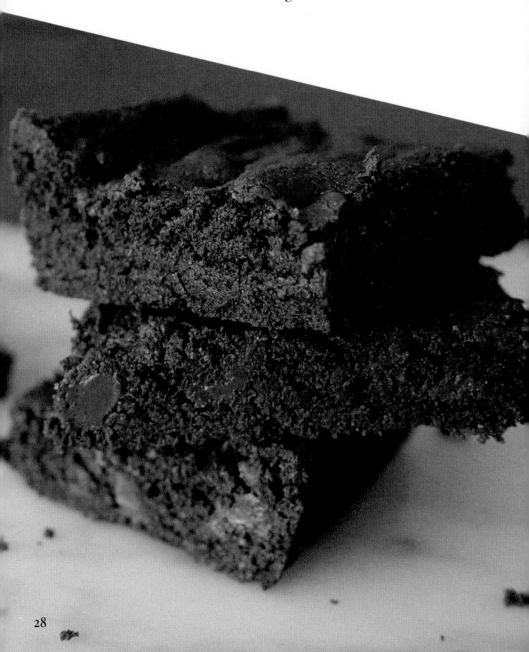

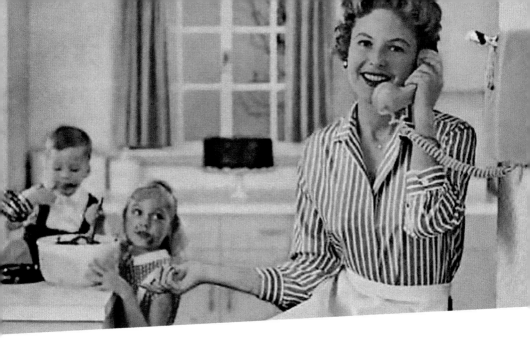

1 tablespoon non-hydrogenated vegetable shortening

1/4 cup water

1/4 cup all-purpose flour

3/4 cup sugar

1 teaspoon vanilla

1/2 cup non-dairy butter, melted

3/4 cup unsweetened cocoa powder

2/3 cup unsifted whole-wheat pastry flour

2 1/4 teaspoons baking powder, separated

1/4 teaspoon salt

1/2 cup non-dairy semi-sweet chocolate chips

yield: 16 brownies

1. Preheat the oven to 350 degrees. Grease a 8x8-inch baking pan.

2. In a medium bowl, combine the shortening, water, all-purpose flour, and 1 teaspoon of baking powder. Blend in the sugar and vanilla; add the butter.

3. Gradually combine the dry ingredients to the wet mixture. Fold in the chocolate chips.

4. Scoop the batter and spread evenly into your baking pan. Bake for 20 minutes. Cool.

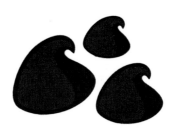

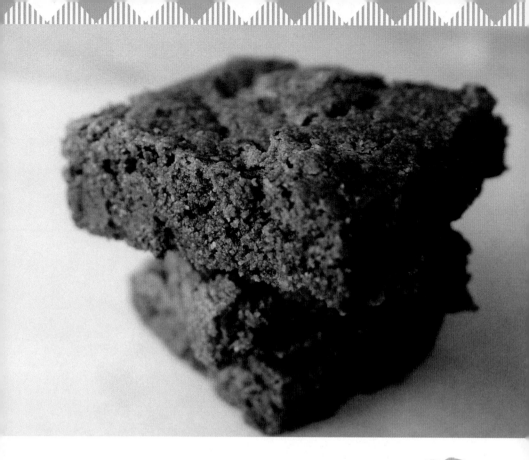

S ome recipes are more challenging than others, and this
one was definitely a challenge but well worth the effort.
I have always loved a blondie and was determined to
make a great one without eggs. However, that goal was easier
said than done.

I quickly learned that the interplay between certain
combinations of ingredients was particularly difficult
with this dessert. There was a lengthy trial-and-error
process behind this bar cookie, until I finally realized
the winning combination of oat flour and coconut
sugar. The oat flour paired with coconut sugar gives
this blondie not only stability but also its distinctive
caramel color and smooth flavor.

blondies (Gluten Free)

This blondie is revised from Ruth Wakefield's original 1930's Toll House Cookie recipe. A lighter version of the classic chocolate brownie, this blondie holds its own.

yield: 16 blondies

2 cups oat flour, sifted

1/2 teaspoon baking soda

1/2 teaspoon salt

1/3 cup non-dairy butter, softened

1/3 cup non-hydrogenated vegetable shortening

1 cup coconut sugar

1 tablespoon ground flaxseed mixed in 3 tablespoons water (let sit 5 minutes)

8 ounces (1 1/4 cups) non-dairy semi-sweet chocolate chips

1. Preheat the oven to 350 degrees. Grease a 8x8-inch baking pan.

2. In a small bowl, sift the flour, baking soda and salt.

3. In a separate large bowl, cream the non-dairy butter, vegetable shortening, coconut sugar, and vanilla extract together until smooth. Add the flaxseed mixture.

4. Gradually incorporate the flour mixture and blend well.

5. Fold in the chocolate chips and transfer the batter to your baking pan.

6. Bake for 20 to 25 minutes and cool completely before cutting into squares.

s'mores

My version of this campfire classic was inspired by the first official S'mores recipe that was published in the Girl Scout's Handbook back in 1927.

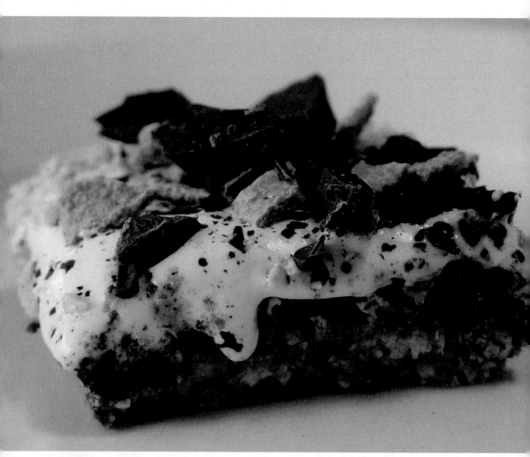

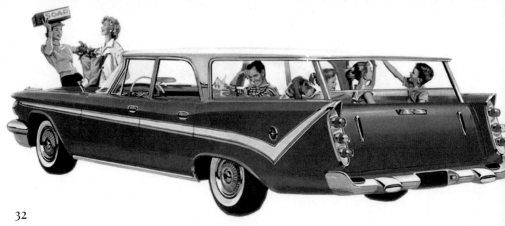

yield: 24 bars

for the crust

2 1/4 cups graham cracker crumbs

3 tablespoons coconut sugar

1/4 teaspoon salt

6 tablespoons non-dairy butter, melted

for the brownies

6 ounces non-dairy semi-sweet chocolate, chopped

3/4 cup non-dairy butter, softened

1/2 cup water plus 1 tablespoon mixed with 3 tablespoons ground flaxseed (let sit 5 minutes)

1 1/4 cups coconut sugar

1 cup all-purpose flour

1 teaspoon salt

2 teaspoons vanilla

for the topping:

1-7.5 ounce jar of marshmallow cream

2 tablespoons hemp milk

3 whole graham cracker boards, chopped up

1/2 cup chopped non-dairy semi-sweet chocolate pieces

directions for crust:

1. Preheat the oven to 350 degrees.

2. Combine 2 1/4 cups of graham cracker crumbs, sugar, salt, and butter in a bowl until evenly moistened.

3. Scoop into a 13x9x2-inch baking pan; press evenly into the bottom.

4. Refrigerate for one hour or until set.

directions for brownie:

5. Combine the semi-sweet chocolate and butter in a microwave-proof bowl and heat in 30-second intervals until softened. Stir until smooth; let cool.

6. In a large bowl, combine the flaxseed mixture, coconut sugar, and vanilla, and mix well; add the cooled chocolate mixture. Stir in the flour and salt and mix until combined.

7. Pour over crust and spread evenly. Bake at 350 degrees for 30 minutes or until a toothpick inserted in the center comes out clean.

directions for topping:

8. Whisk marshmallow cream and hemp milk in a medium bowl until smooth.

9. Pour the marshmallow cream over the top of the brownie, tilting the pan to spread evenly.

10. Sprinkle with chopped graham crackers and chocolate pieces.

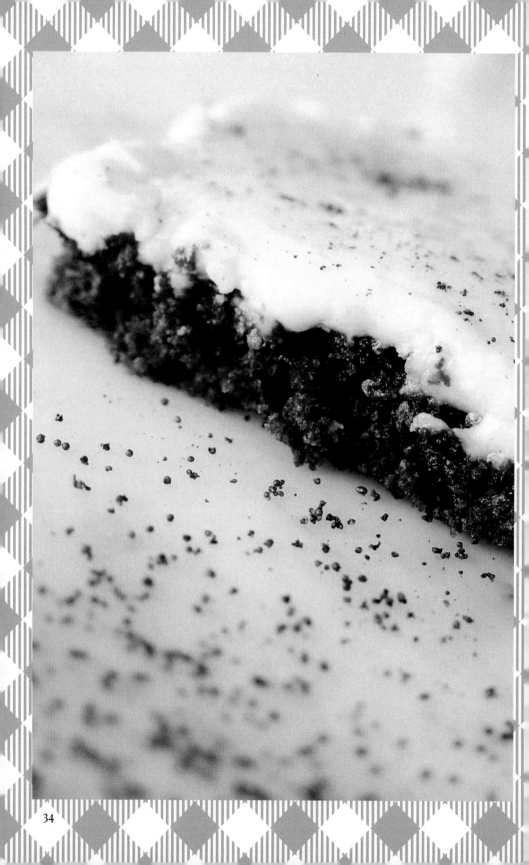

molasses creams

Adapted from the Farm Journal's Country Cookbook, *dated 1959, these wonderful frosted bars have just the right amount of spice to make them a traditional favorite.*

yield: 18 bars

1/2 cup non-hydrogenated vegetable shortening

1/2 cup sugar

1 tablespoon ground flaxseed mixed in 3 tablespoons water (let sit for 5 minutes)

1/2 cup molasses

1/3 cup strong coffee, hot

1 1/2 cups sifted spelt flour

1 1/2 teaspoons baking powder

3/4 teaspoon salt

1/4 teaspoon baking soda

1 teaspoon cinnamon

1/2 teaspoon ground cloves

Instant espresso coffee for garnish

for the frosting:

1/4 cup non-dairy butter

2 cups confectioners sugar

2 tablespoons coffee

1. Preheat the oven to 350 degrees.

2. Cream the shortening and sugar; blend in the flaxseed mixture, molasses, and coffee.

3. Sift together the remaining ingredients and add to the wet ingredients; blend well.

4. Pour into a greased 9x13-inch pan. Bake for 25 minutes.

directions for frosting:

5. Cream the butter with the confectioners sugar and add the coffee; mix until smooth enough to spread.

6. Frost the bars while still warm. Cool completely and then sprinkle with instant espresso coffee.

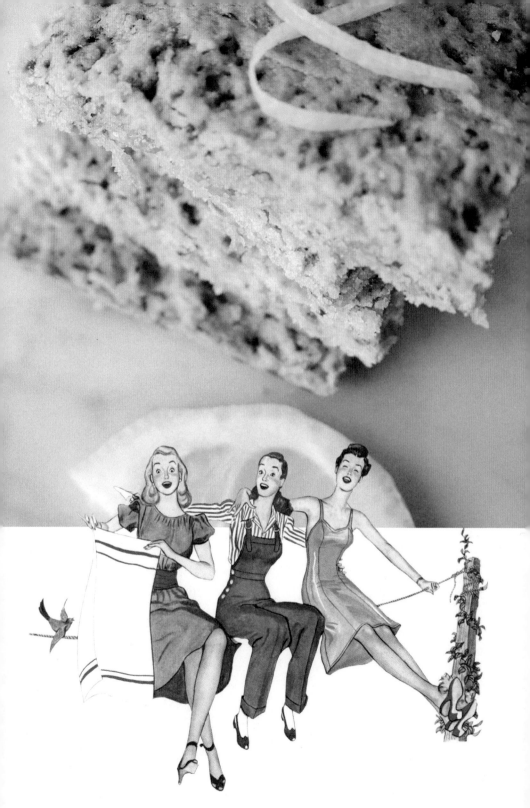

lemon cake bars

This light, fresh cake bar brings me back to long summer days spent at the beach and picnic lunches. Revised from the CIA *Encyclopedic Cookbook, dated 1950.*

yield: 35 two-inch squares

1 ³/₄ cups plus 4 teaspoons all-purpose flour

1/4 cup cornstarch

1/4 teaspoon salt

1 teaspoon baking powder

1/3 cup non-hydrogenated vegetable shortening

3/4 coconut sugar

1 tablespoon ground flaxseed mixed with 3 tablespoons of water

1/3 cup plus 2 tablespoons almond milk

2 tablespoons lemon juice

2 tablespoons lemon zest

1. Preheat the oven to 350 degrees. Grease a 15x10x1-inch sheet pan.

2. Cream the shortening, add the coconut sugar and mix thoroughly; add the flaxseed mixture.

3. Sift the dry ingredients together and add to the creamed mixture alternately with the almond milk and the lemon juice. Fold in the lemon zest.

4. Bake for about 20 minutes. Cool.

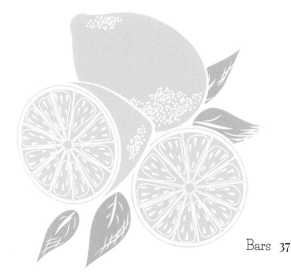

fudge squares

You can never have enough chocolate. These flavorful squares are lighter than traditional chocolate brownies. This recipe was revised from Pillsbury's Best of the Bake-off Collection, *dated 1959.*

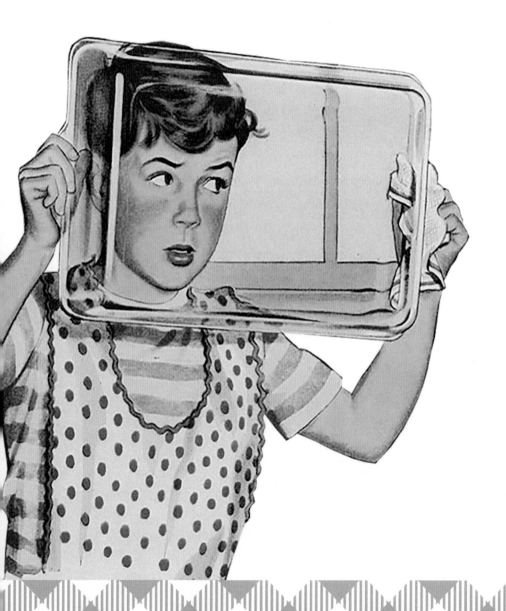

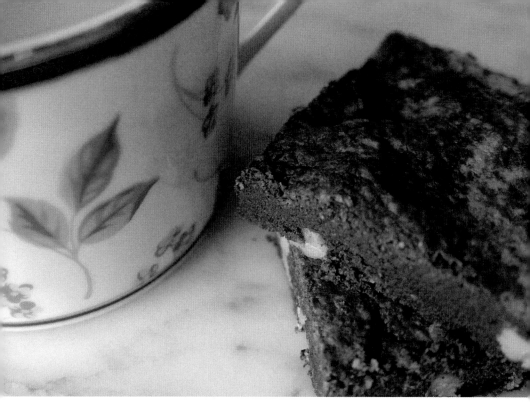

yield: 30 two-inch bars

6 ounces of chopped non-dairy semi-sweet chocolate

1/2 cup non-dairy butter

3/4 cup coconut sugar

1 teaspoon vanilla

1 1/2 cups sifted flour

1 teaspoon baking powder

1/2 teaspoon salt

3/4 cup chopped walnuts

1. Preheat the oven to 350 degrees. Grease a 9x13x2-inch baking pan.

2. In a microwave-safe bowl, melt the chocolate in 30-second intervals until smooth.

3. In a medium-sized bowl, cream together the butter, coconut sugar, and vanilla.

4. In a separate bowl, sift the flour, baking powder, and salt together. Stir into the creamed mixture; mix in the melted chocolate and nuts.

5. Press the dough (will be thick and crumbly) into an ungreased 9x13-inch baking pan; bake for 18 to 20 minutes. Cool.

CAKES

vanilla doughnuts

Instead of deep frying, here is a wholesome version of the classic buttermilk doughnut revised from Grandma Kay's 1954 Westinghouse Cookbook; these are great served for breakfast.

yield: about 18 mini-doughnuts

1 1/4 cups oat flour

1/2 teaspoon baking soda

1/4 teaspoon salt

1/2 cup oat milk plus
1 teaspoon lemon juice (mix
and let sit 10 minutes)

1/3 cup packed brown sugar

3 tablespoons aquafaba

4 teaspoons non-dairy
butter, melted

1 teaspoon vanilla extract

1. Preheat the oven to 325 degrees. Coat mini-doughnut pan with non-stick cooking spray.

2. In a large bowl, mix the flour, baking soda, and salt.

3. In a smaller bowl, whisk the oat milk mixture, sugar, aquafaba, butter, and vanilla until smooth. Add the milk mixture to the dry ingredients and mix well.

4. Spoon batter into a large resealable bag, cut off corner. Squeeze batter into doughnut molds and fill 2/3.

5. Smooth tops and bake for 5 to 10 minutes or until tops spring back when touched. Remove from pan promptly and cool on a rack.

Tip: Try drizzling both the chocolate and white icings on these doughnuts (the recipe for white icing is listed under chocolate doughnuts).

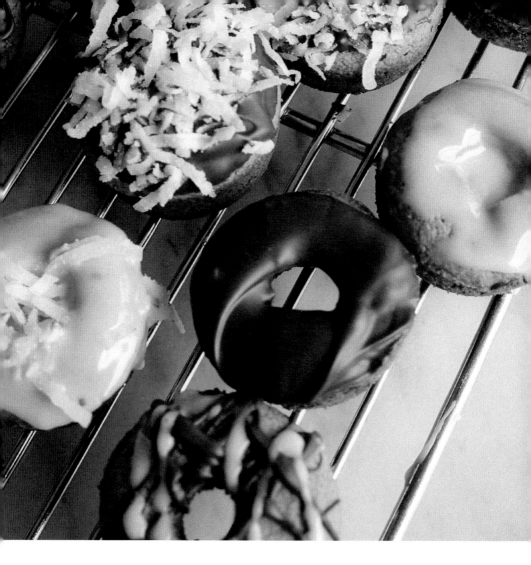

for chocolate icing:

1 cup of confectioners sugar

2 tablespoons oat milk

1 tablespoon unsweetened cocoa powder

Shredded coconut for topping

1. In a medium-sized bowl, combine the confectioners sugar, cocoa, and oat milk. Stir until smooth.

2. Dip cooled doughnuts into the bowl and allow the excess icing to drip back into the bowl.

3. Place doughnuts on the rack and top with shredded coconut.

chocolate doughnuts

These little chocolate goodies will be gone as soon as you make them. Get out your mini-doughnut pan for these scrumptious treats revised from the 1954 Westinghouse Cookbook.

yield: about 18 mini doughnuts

1 cup all-purpose flour

1/4 cup unsweetened cocoa powder

1/2 teaspoon baking soda

1/4 teaspoon salt

1/2 cup oat milk plus
1 teaspoon lemon juice
(mix and let sit 10 minutes)

1/2 cup packed brown sugar

3 tablespoons aquafaba

4 teaspoons non-dairy butter, melted

1 teaspoon vanilla extract

1. Preheat the oven to 325 degrees. Coat a mini-doughnut pan with non-stick cooking spray.

2. In a large bowl, mix the flour, cocoa powder, baking soda, and salt.

3. In a smaller bowl, whisk the oat milk mixture, sugar, aquafaba, butter, and vanilla until smooth. Add the milk mixture to the dry ingredients and incorporate well.

4. Spoon batter into a large resealable bag, cut off the corner and squeeze into mini-doughnut mold, 2/3 full.

5. Smooth tops and bake from 5 to 10 minutes or until tops spring back when touched. Remove doughnuts from the pan and cool on a rack.

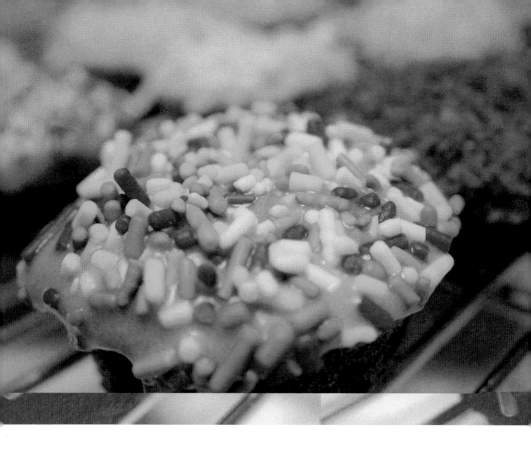

for white icing:

1 cup of confectioners sugar

1 tablespoon oat milk

Sprinkles, shaved non-dairy semi-sweet chocolate for toppings

1. In a medium-sized bowl, combine the confectioners sugar and oat milk. Stir until smooth.

2. Dip cooled doughnuts into the bowl and allow the excess icing to drip back into the bowl.

3. Place doughnuts back on rack and top with shaved chocolate or sprinkles.

Tip: Try this peanut butter glaze: mix 1-1/2 tablespoons water, 2/3 cup powdered sugar, and 1 tablespoon creamy peanut butter until smooth; drizzle on doughnuts.

chocolate cake

Chocolate cake was a favorite in our family and my mom didn't celebrate a birthday without one. This moist and rich cake was revised from Hershey's 1934 Cookbook.

yield: 8 slices

1 ½ cups all-purpose flour

1/2 cup whole-wheat pastry flour

3/4 cup unsweentened cocoa powder

1 ½ teaspoons baking soda

1 teaspoon baking powder

Pinch of salt

1/2 cup of coconut oil

3/4 cup coconut sugar

1 cup plus 2 tablespoons maple syrup

1 cup oat milk mixed with 2 tablespoons chocolate syrup

1 teaspoon vanilla extract

1 teaspoon apple cider vinegar

1. Preheat the oven to 350 degrees. Grease two 9-inch cake pans and line bottoms with parchment paper.

2. Sift the flours, cocoa, baking soda, baking powder, and salt together in a large bowl.

3. With a mixer, combine the coconut oil and coconut sugar together in another large bowl; beat on low for about two minutes. Add maple syrup until combined; add chocolate-oat milk, vanilla extract, and apple cider vinegar, and beat until fully incorporated.

4. Add wet ingredients to dry ingredients; fold with spatula until batter is smooth.

5. Divide batter between cake pans and spread tops to level.

6. Bake until tops spring back, about 30 minutes. Remove pans from oven and cool completely before frosting.

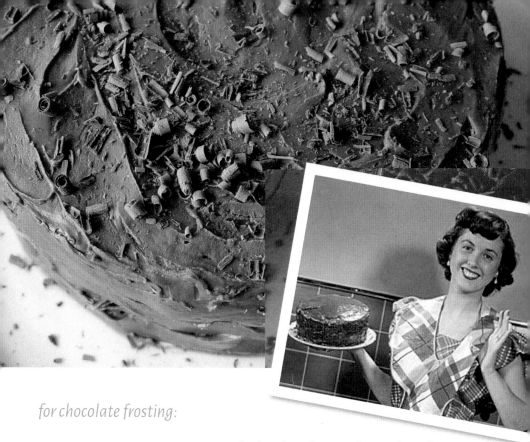

for chocolate frosting:

6 ounces non-dairy semi-sweet, chocolate

4 tablespoons non-dairy butter

5 $\frac{1}{2}$ cups of confectioners sugar, sifted

1/2 teaspoon salt

2 teaspoons vanilla

12 tablespoons oat milk

1. Melt the **chocolate and non-dairy butter in a** microwave-safe bowl in 30-second intervals until smooth.

2. Alternate by adding the confectioners sugar and oat milk to the chocolate mixture, mixing well with each addition.

3. Continue alternating the confectioners sugar with the oat milk until all of the oat milk is added and the frosting is of spreadable consistency. You may not need to add all of the confectioners sugar.

Tip: If the frosting is too stiff, add a little more oat milk, 1 teaspoon at a time; if it's too wet, add more powdered sugar, 1/8 cup at a time.

pineapple cake

This classic pineapple upside-down cake recipe, revised from Marguerite Patten's Every Day Cookbook, *from 1968, gets its dark caramel-glazed pineapples from the addition of coconut sugar.*

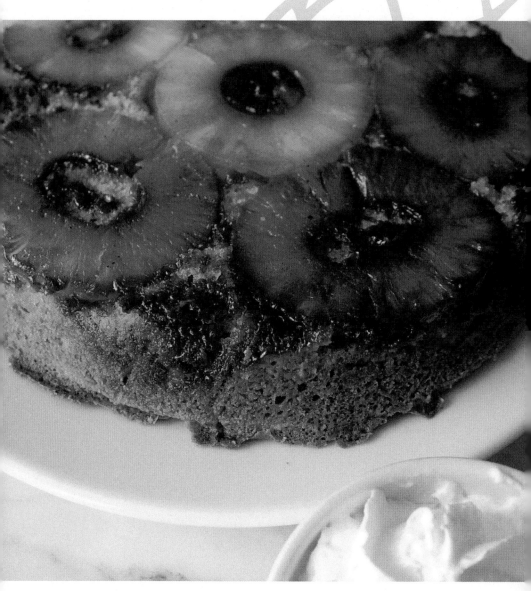

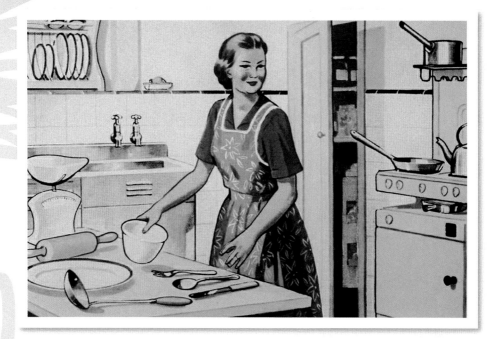

yield: 8 slices

6 tablespoons aquafaba

1/4 cup no-taste vegetable oil

1/2 cup maple syrup

1 cup pineapple juice

2 teaspoons vanilla

1 cup oat flour

1 cup whole-wheat pastry flour

4 teaspoons baking powder

Pinch of salt

1/4 cup coconut oil

1/4 cup coconut sugar

6 canned pineapple rings, reserve juice

1. Preheat the oven to 350 degrees. Oil and flour the sides of an 8x8-inch round cake pan.

2. Whisk the aquafaba, oil, syrup, and juice together.

3. In a separate bowl, mix the flours, baking powder, and salt. Add the wet ingredients to the dry and mix well.

4. In a separate microwave-safe bowl, melt the coconut oil, and stir in the coconut sugar until smooth.

5. Pour liquid into the bottom of the cake pan.

6. Line the bottom of pan with the pineapple rings.

7. Pour the batter over the pineapple and bake for 30 to 40 minutes.

lemon cake

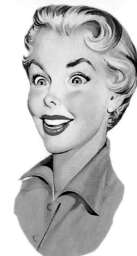

Adapted from Good Housekeeping's 1930s Meals Tested, Tasted, and Approved Cookbook, this light and lemony version of a torte pairs wonderfully with a rich meal.

yield: 8 slices

1 cup whole-wheat pastry flour

1 cup all-purpose flour

1 teaspoon baking powder

1 teaspoons baking soda

1 tablespoon lemon zest

1/3 cup canola oil

3/4 cup maple syrup

2/3 cup oat milk

1/4 cup lemon juice

1/3 cup water

1 teaspoon salt

1 teaspoon vanilla extract

2 teaspoons lemon extract

1. Preheat the oven to 350 degrees. Oil and lightly flour two 8-inch cake pans.

2. Sift the flours, baking powder, and baking soda into a large bowl. Add the lemon zest and mix with a wire whisk to combine.

3. In a medium bowl, combine the remaining ingredients and add to the flour mixture, incorporating well.

4. Pour batter evenly into prepared pans. Bake for 20 minutes or until the cake springs back when lightly pressed. Be careful not to over bake. These layers will be thin. Cool completely before frosting.

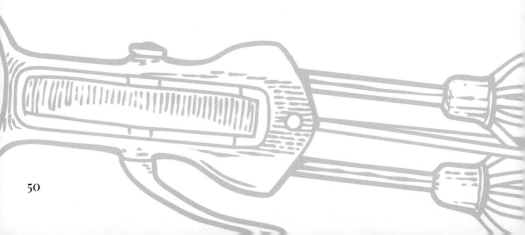

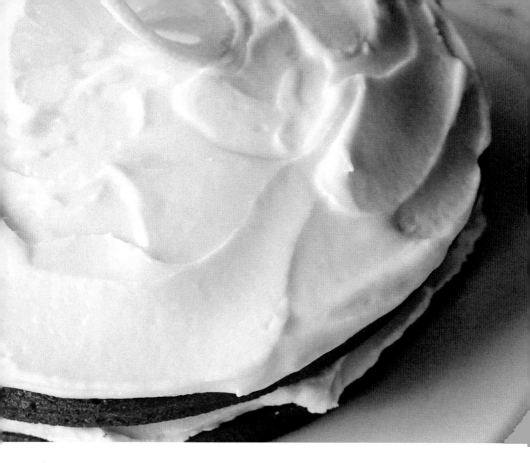

for lemon frosting:

4 cups confectioners sugar

6 tablespoons
non-dairy butter

4 teaspoons lemon extract

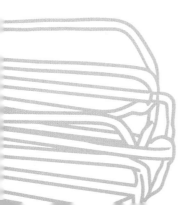

1. Cream the non-dairy butter and lemon extract together in a large bowl.

2. Gradually add the confectioners sugar, beating well with each addition. Continue until all of the sugar is added and the mixture reaches spreading consistency.

3. Place the bottom layer of cake on a cake plate. Frost the top of the bottom layer right up to the edges of the cake.

4. Place the second cake on top of the frosted layer. Frost the top of the second layer, spreading the frosting to the edges of the cake.

coffee cake

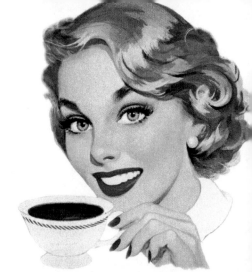

*Every baker has their own version
of this cake. Mine is adapted from*
American Woman's Cookbook,
*dated 1962, with the addition of
pumpkin, spice, and a crumb topping.*

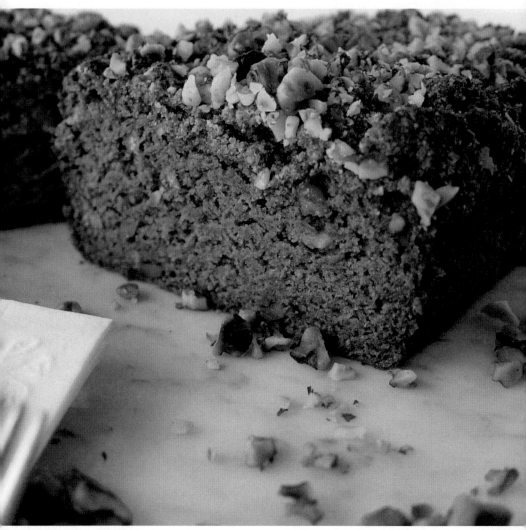

yield: 12 slices

3/4 cup spelt flour

3/4 cup oat flour

2 teaspoons baking powder

1 teaspoon cinnamon

1/4 teaspoon ground nutmeg

1/4 teaspoon ground, dried ginger

1/8 teaspoon ground cloves

1/2 teaspoon salt

3 tablespoons aquafaba

1/2 cup coconut sugar

1 cup canned pumpkin, packed

1/4 cup vegetable oil

1 teaspoon vanilla

1/2 cup chopped walnuts

for crumb topping:

1/4 cup non-dairy butter, softened

1/3 cup coconut sugar, packed

1/2 cup spelt flour

1/3 cup of walnuts, chopped fine

1. Preheat the oven to 350 degrees. Grease a 9x5x3-inch loaf pan.

2. Mix the flours, baking powder, spices, and salt in a large bowl.

3. Beat the aquafaba and coconut sugar in a medium bowl and add the pumpkin, oil, and vanilla. Mix until smooth.

4. Gradually add the wet ingredients to the dry and stir until just moistened and the batter comes together.

5. Fold in walnuts and spoon batter into pan.

directions for crumb topping:

6. Cream the butter and coconut sugar together.

7. Add the flour and stir until crumbly. Mix in the walnuts.

8. Sprinkle over the batter and bake for about 50 minutes. Cool completely on rack before slicing.

carrot cake

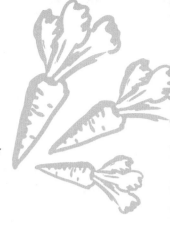

The all-night diners in New Jersey along Route 17 used to serve carrot cake with fluffy white frosting 24/7. Adapted from the Encyclopedia of Cookery Cookbook, *dated 1949.*

serves 8-10

2 cups all-purpose flour

1 tablespoon baking powder

1 teaspoon ground cinnamon

1 teaspoon ground nutmeg

1/2 teaspoon salt

4 tablespoons ground flaxseeds mixed in 3/4 cup water

1 cup vegetable oil

2 cups sugar

3 cups shredded or julienned carrots

1 cup chopped pecans

1. Preheat the oven to 350 degrees. Grease an 11x9-inch baking pan.

2. In a large bowl, stir together the oil, sugar, carrots, walnuts, flour, baking powder, cinnamon, nutmeg, and salt.

3. Add the flaxseed mixture and mix well.

4. Pour the batter into the prepared pan and bake until the cake springs back when lightly touched, about 45 minutes.

5. Cool completely before frosting.

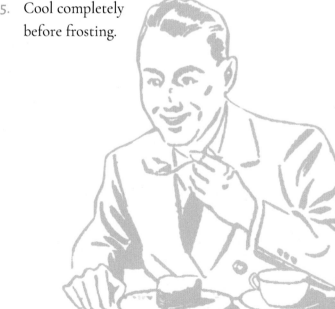

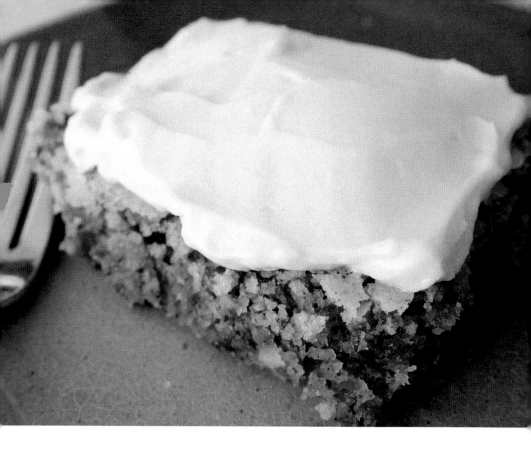

for frosting:

1 1/2 cups confectioners sugar

4 tablespoons non-dairy butter, softened

1/4 cup non-hydrogenated vegetable shortening

12 ounces vegan cream cheese

1 tablespoon vanilla

2 tablespoons oat milk

1. Beat the butter, shortening, and cream cheese together until smooth.

2. Gradually add the confectioners sugar, alternating with the vanilla extract and oat milk.

3. Blend until the frosting reaches spreading consistency.

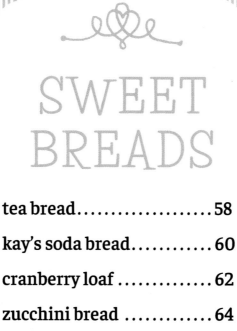

SWEET BREADS

tea bread

We made this cake bread in my Little Chefs cooking class and it was a hit; they loved the chocolate and you will too! Revised from Hershey's Cookbook, *dated 1962.*

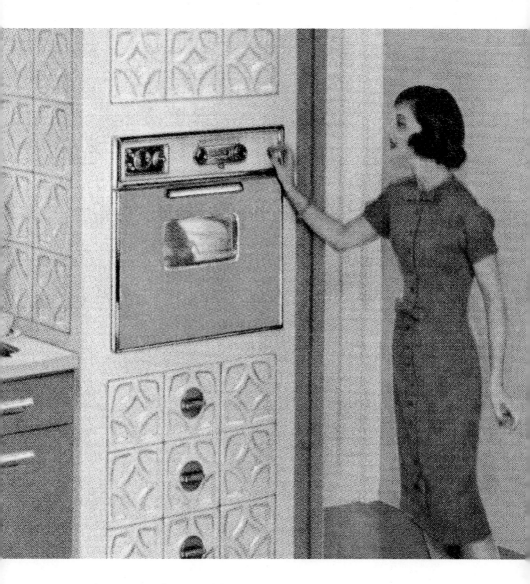

Tip: Don't have cake flour? Add 2 tablespoons of cornstarch to a 1 cup dry measure, then fill in the cup with all-purpose flour and level off.

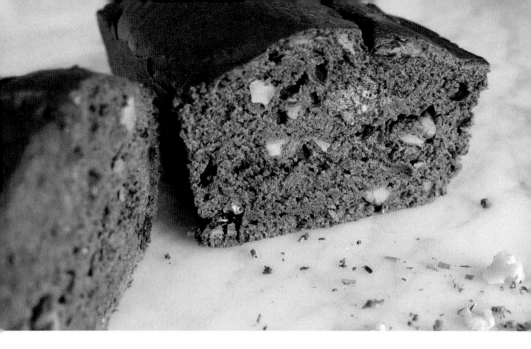

yield: 12 slices

1/4 cup non-dairy butter, softened

2/3 cup coconut sugar

1 tablespoon ground flax seed mixed with 3 tablespoons water

2 cups cake flour, sifted (see tip)

1 teaspoon baking soda

3/4 teaspoon salt

1/3 cup cocoa powder

1 cup oat milk plus 1 tablespoon white vinegar (let sit for 10 minutes)

1 cup non-dairy semi-sweet chocolate, chopped

3/4 cup walnuts, chopped

1. Preheat the oven to 350 degrees. Grease a 9x5x2-inch loaf pan.

2. Cream the non-dairy butter and add the coconut sugar a little at a time, mixing well with each addition. Add the flaxseed mixture and beat well.

3. Sift the flour, baking soda, salt, and cocoa powder.

4. Add the flour mixture to the wet ingredients, alternating with the oat milk, stirring until well blended.

5. Stir in the chocolate and walnuts.

6. Bake for 1 hour. Completely cool before slicing.

kay's soda bread

I always use currants instead of raisins when making this very special recipe, revised from Grandma Kay's little recipe box dating back to the 1940s.

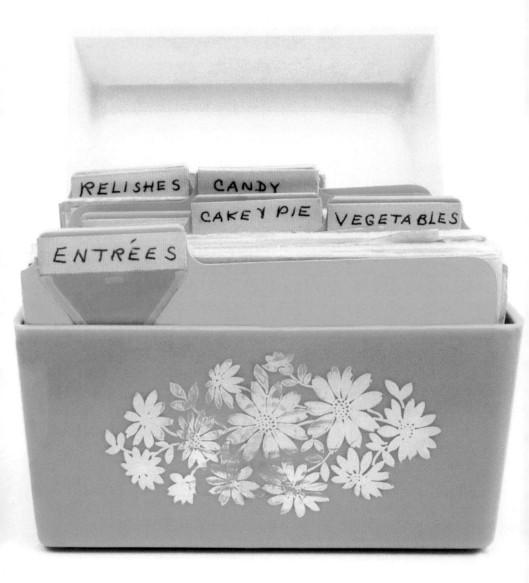

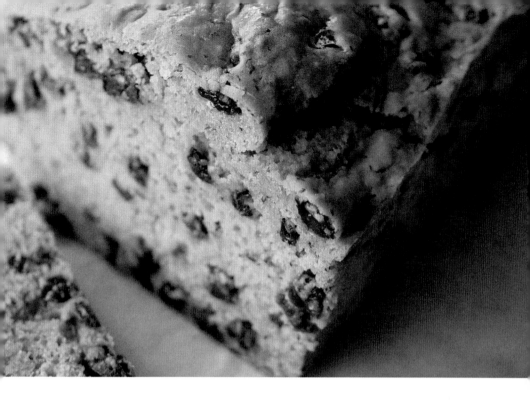

serves 12

3 cups all-purpose flour, sifted

2/3 cup coconut sugar

3 teaspoons baking powder

1 teaspoon baking soda

1 teaspoon salt

1 1/2 cups currants

2 tablespoons ground flaxseed mixed with 6 tablespoons water

2 cups cashew milk mixed with 2 tablespoons white vinegar (let sit for 10 minutes)

2 tablespoons butter, melted

1. Preheat the oven to 350 degrees. Grease a 9x5x2-inch loaf pan.

2. Mix the flour, sugar, baking powder, baking soda, and salt together. Stir in the currants.

3. Combine the remaining ingredients and add to the dry mixture. Mix until the flour is just moistened.

4. Turn batter into loaf pan and bake for 1 hour or until tooth pick inserted in the middle comes out clean.

5. Cool completely before serving.

cranberry loaf

Thanksgiving Day begins with a toasted slice of this bread and a strong cup of black coffee. Revised from Good Housekeeping's Breads & Sandwiches Cookbook, *dated 1958.*

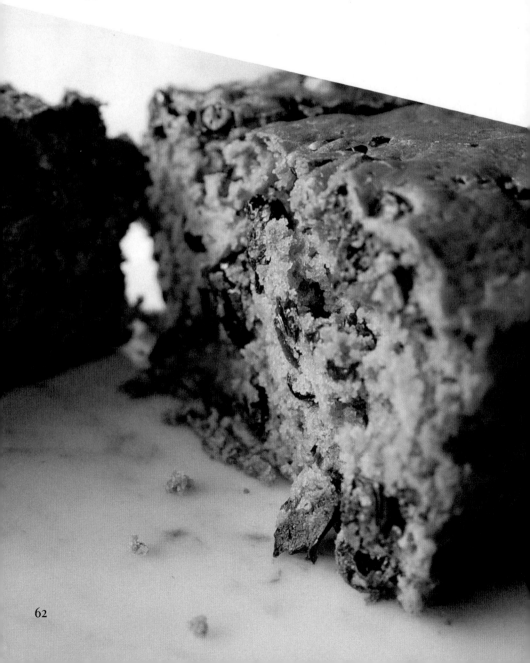

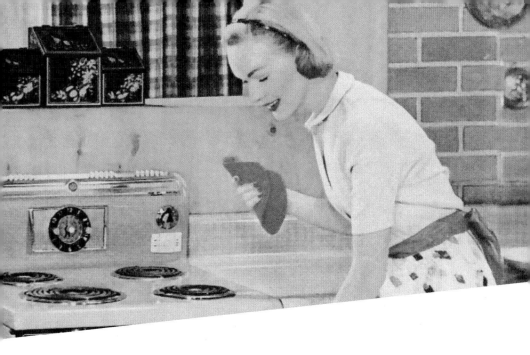

serves 12

2 cups all-purpose
flour, sifted

1 cup coconut sugar

1 ¹/₂ teaspoons
baking powder

1/2 teaspoon baking soda

1 teaspoon salt

1/4 cup coconut oil

1 tablespoon ground flax
seeds mixed with
3 tablespoons water

1 teaspoon grated
orange peel

3/4 cup orange juice

1 ¹/₂ cups raisins

1 ¹/₂ cups dried cranberries

1. Preheat the oven to 350 degrees. Grease a 9x5x2-inch loaf pan.

2. Sift the flour, sugar, baking powder, baking soda, and salt together in a large bowl. Cut in the coconut oil and stir until the mixture is crumbly.

3. Combine the remaining wet ingredients and add to the dry mixture; mix until flour is moistened. Fold in the fruit.

4. Scoop batter into loaf pan and bake for 50 minutes or until a toothpick inserted in the middle comes out clean.

5. Cool completely before slicing.

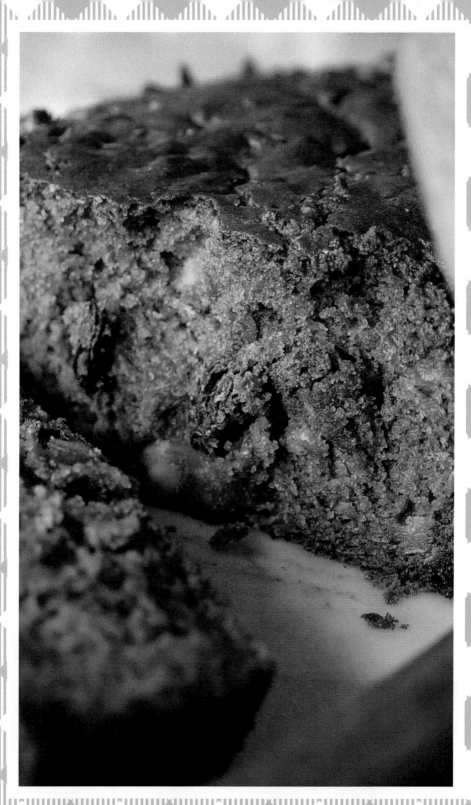

zucchini bread

Gluten Free

I adapted this recipe from McCall's Cookbook, dated 1963. The unique combination of zucchini and select spices make a bread that pairs well with just about any meal.

serves 12

1 ½ cups quinoa flour

1 teaspoon baking powder

1 teaspoon baking soda

1/2 teaspoon salt

1 teaspoon cinnamon

1/2 cup vegetable oil

4 ½ tablespoons aquafaba

1 cup coconut sugar

1 teaspoon vanilla

1 cup grated zucchini

1/4 cup raisins

1/4 cup chopped walnuts

1. Preheat the oven to 325 degrees. Grease a 9x5x2-inch loaf pan.

2. Sift the flour, baking powder, baking soda, and spices together in a large bowl.

3. In another bowl, blend the oil, aquafaba, sugar, and vanilla together.

4. Gradually add to the dry mixture until the flour is just moistened. Fold in the zucchini, raisins, and walnuts.

5. Spoon into prepared pan. Bake for 1 hour. Cool.

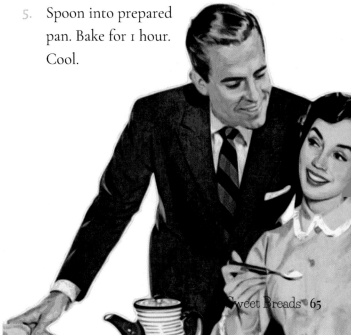

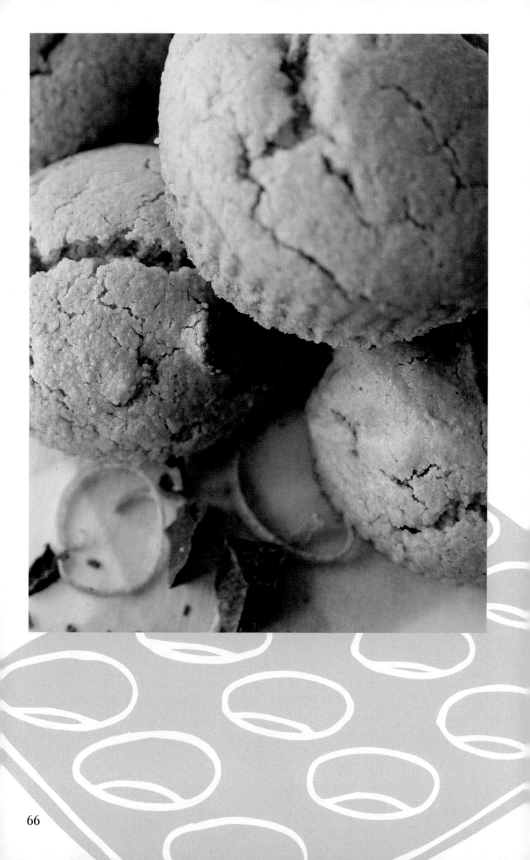

chocolate chip muffins

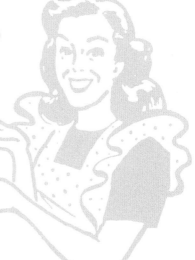

These muffins serve well when toasted; brightly flavored orange zest compliments the full-bodied dark chocolate in this revised recipe from Betty Crocker's Picture Cookbook, *dated 1961.*

makes 1 dozen muffins

1 1/2 cups all-purpose flour

2 teaspoons baking powder

1/2 teaspoon salt

1/2 cup coconut sugar

1/2 cup oat milk

1/4 cup vegetable oil

3 tablespoons aquafaba

1 teaspoon orange zest

3/4 cup non-dairy semi-sweet chocolate chips

1. Preheat the oven to 375 degrees. Grease or line muffin tins.

2. Mix the flour, baking powder, and salt together in a large bowl.

3. In another bowl, blend the sugar, oat milk, oil, and aquafaba together.

4. Gradually add to the dry mixture until the flour is just moistened. Fold in the zest and chocolate chips.

5. Spoon batter into prepared muffin tins, about 2/3 full.

6. Bake for 15 to 20 minutes.

pumpkin muffins

These muffins are great when served for breakfast or with dinner. Adapted from The Art of Cooking and Serving Cookbook, *dated 1937.*

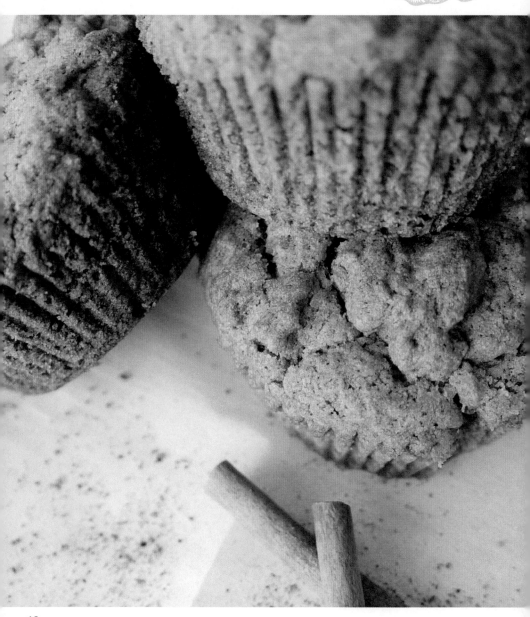

1/2 cup canned pumpkin

1 cup vegetable oil

1 cup coconut sugar

2 cups all-purpose flour

2 teaspoons baking powder

1 teaspoon baking soda

1 teaspoon salt

1/2 teaspoon cinnamon

1/2 teaspoon nutmeg

1/4 teaspoon mace

6 tablespoons aquafaba

1. Preheat the oven to 350 degrees. Grease or line muffin tins.

2. Sift the flour, baking powder, baking soda, salt, and spices together in a large bowl.

3. Mix the pumpkin, oil, and sugar together well.

4. Add the aquafaba and then the dry ingredients gradually, mixing after each addition.

5. Spoon the batter into tins.

6. Bake for 20 to 25 minutes.

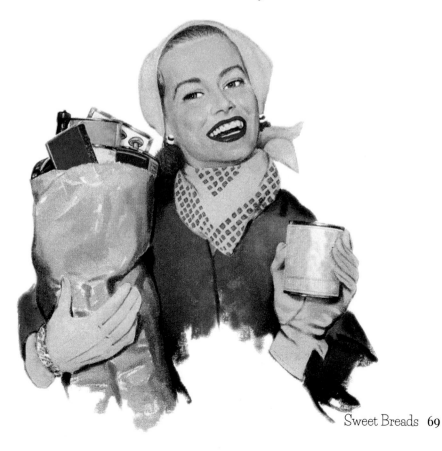

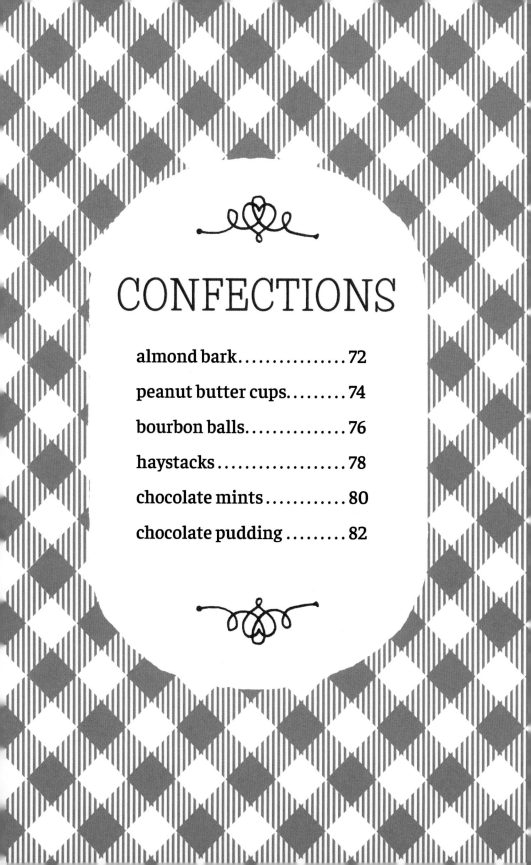

CONFECTIONS

almond bark

Gluten Free

This bark reminds me of a Hershey's Bar with Almonds. Hershey's first chocolate bar came out in 1900 and has been a staple in American culture ever since. Adapted from Hershey's Cookbook, dated 1934.

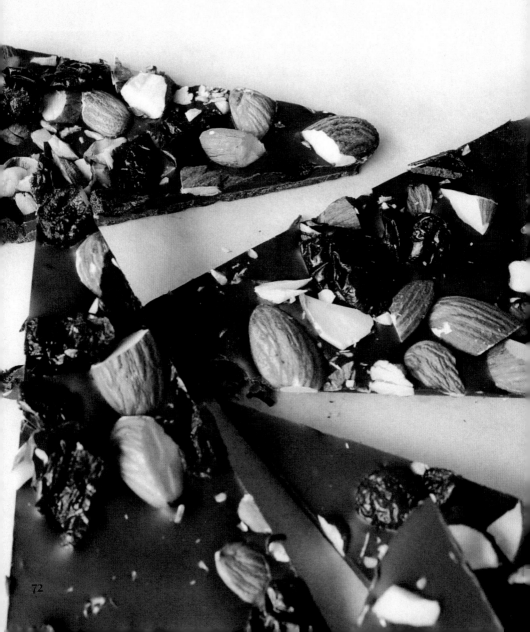

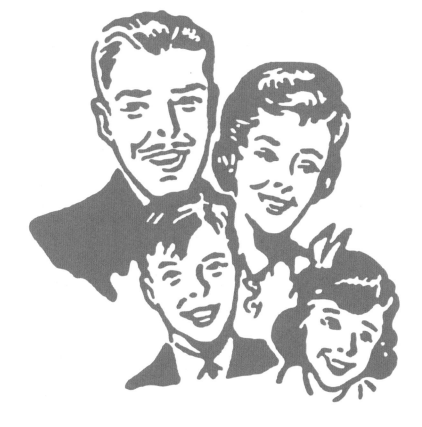

12 ounces of non-dairy semi-sweet chocolate, roughly chopped

1 cup almonds, roughly chopped

1 cup dried cranberries

1. Line a cookie sheet with parchment paper.

2. Place the chopped chocolate in a microwave-safe bowl and heat 2 minutes. Continue heating in 30-second intervals until melted. Stir until smooth.

3. Pour chocolate onto parchment-lined cookie sheet.

4. Sprinkle with the cranberries and almonds; gently press the almonds and cranberries into the chocolate.

5. Chill for 2 hours or until set.

6. Break into pieces and store in a cool place.

peanut butter cups

Gluten Free

Reeses's Peanut Butter Cups have been around since 1928. This recipe revised from The Toll House Heritage Cookbook, dated 1934, uses only pure, non-processed ingredients.

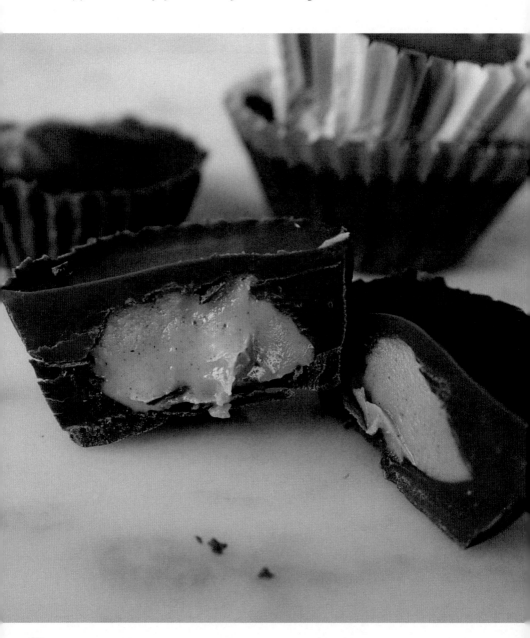

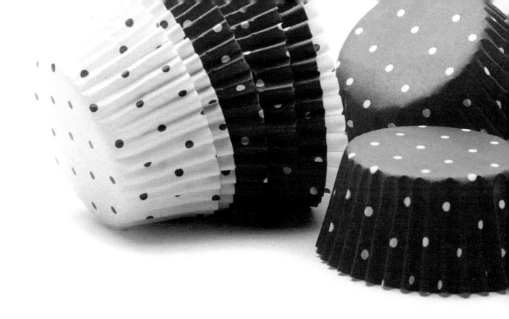

yield: two dozen peanut butter cups

12 ounces of non-dairy
semi-sweet chocolate,
roughly chopped

2 tablespoons non-
hydrogenated vegetable
shortening

1/2 cup no-stir, non-
hydrogenated creamy
peanut butter

24-1 1/4 inch
paper candy cups

*Tip: For Mallow
Cups, substitute
marshmallow cream
for the peanut butter.*

1. Line a cookie sheet with parchment paper.
    Place 24 candy cups on top of the
    parchment paper.

2. In a microwave-safe bowl, heat the chocolate
    and shortening for 2 minutes; stir.
    Continue in 30-second intervals until melted;
    stir smooth.

3. Using a teaspoon, pour the melted chocolate
    into the cups lining the bottom.

4. With another teaspoon, place a small dollop
    (about 1/4 to 1/2 teaspoon) of peanut butter
    in the center of the chocolate.

5. Finish by topping the peanut butter with
    another teaspoon of melted chocolate. Chill
    until set, about 1 hour.

6. Store in a cool, dry place.

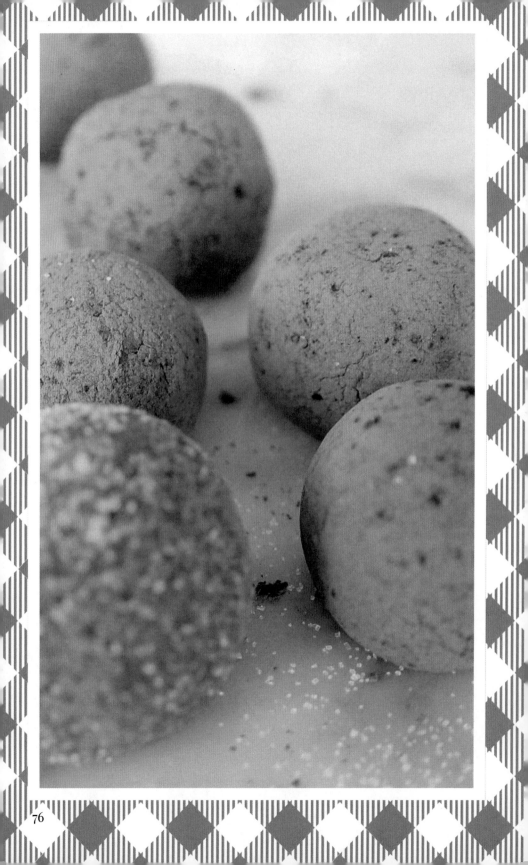

bourbon balls

These candies remind me of my parents' holiday parties. Revised from Betty Crocker's Cooking American Style Cookbook, dated 1975, I use a smooth blended whiskey to give these an extra kick.

makes 5 dozen candies

2 cups vanilla wafer cookies, crushed fine

2 cups pecans, chopped fine

2 cups confectioners sugar

1/4 cup cocoa powder

3/4 cup blended whiskey

1/4 cup corn syrup

Granulated sugar for coating

Cocoa powder for coating

1. Line a cookie sheet with parchment paper.

2. Mix wafers, pecans, sugar, and cocoa. Stir in the whiskey and corn syrup.

3. Shape into 1-inch balls. Roll in granulated sugar or cocoa powder and place onto cookie sheet.

4. Transfer candies to an airtight container and refrigerate for several days before serving.

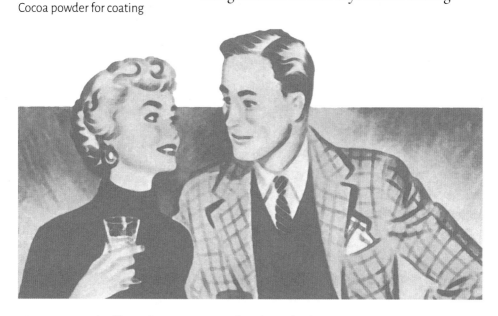

Tip: For rum balls, substitute rum for the whiskey.

haystacks

Haystacks were popular in the 70s. I remember receiving them as a Halloween treat wrapped in waxpaper; this recipe was revised from the 1980 Toll House Heritage Cookbook.

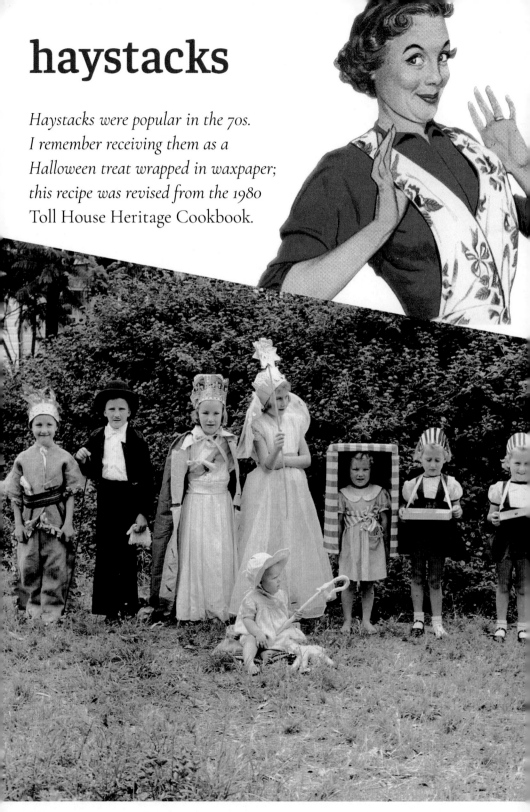

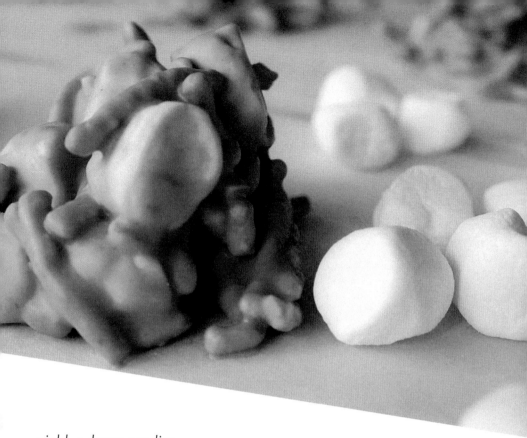

yield: 4 dozen candies

12 ounces all-natural
butterscotch morsels

1 cup non-hydrogenated
peanut butter

1 tablespoon
non-hydrogenated
vegetable shortening

6 ounces of pretzel sticks,
broken

4 cups mini marshmallows

1. In a large microwave-safe bowl, heat the morsels, peanut butter, and shortening in 30-second intervals until fully melted. Stir until smooth.

2. Transfer to a large bowl and fold in the pretzels. Cool for 2 minutes.

3. Fold in marshmallows.

4. Drop by the tablespoon onto parchment-lined cookie sheets and chill until set.

Tip: For Chocolate Haystacks, substitute non-dairy chocolate for the peanut butter, or try fried Chinese noodles instead of pretzels.

chocolate mints

These creamy mints will bring you back to the specialty candy stores that sold hand-made chocolates at reasonable prices; adapted from the Fannie Farmer Cookbook, *dated 1951.*

makes 2 dozen mint candies

12 ounces non-dairy semi-sweet chocolate, roughly chopped and divided

4 tablespoons non-hydrogenated vegetable shortening

for mint filling:

5 tablespoons non-dairy butter

1/2 cup corn syrup

4-1/2 cups confectioners sugar, divided

1 teaspoon peppermint extract

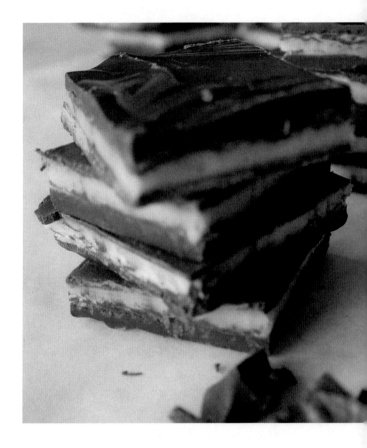

1. Line a 15x10x1-inch cookie sheet with parchment paper.

2. In a microwave-safe bowl, combine 6 ounces of the chopped chocolate and 2 tablespoons shortening and heat until melted; stir until smooth and spread out over parchment paper. Chill until set.

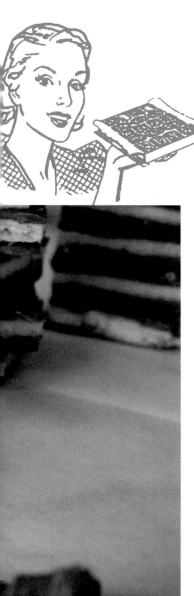

directions for mint filling:

3. Grease a 15x10x1-inch cookie sheet.

4. In a large saucepan, mix the butter, corn syrup, and half of the confectioners sugar; bring to a full boil, stirring continuously over low to medium heat. Add the remaining confectioners sugar and extract; stir vigorously until well blended.

5. Remove from heat. Pour fondant onto greased cookie sheet. Cool for about 5 minutes or until it can be handled.

6. Knead until soft, about 5 minutes.

7. Roll out fondant between 2 sheets of parchment paper to measure a 15x10-inch rectangle about 1/8-inch thick and fit over the bottom layer.

8. Remove the top sheet of parchment paper and invert the fondant over the bottom layer of chocolate.

9. Chill in refrigerator.

directions for top layer

10. In a microwave-safe bowl, melt the remaining chocolate and vegetable shortening together until smooth.

11. Remove parchment paper and spread the chocolate evenly over the mint filling; chill an additional 20 minutes.

12. Cut into 2-inch squares. Store in a cool place.

chocolate pudding

*Adapted from Florence Greenberg's 1951 Cookery Book,
this rich and decadent chocolate pudding is sure to please the
chocolate lover in your family.*

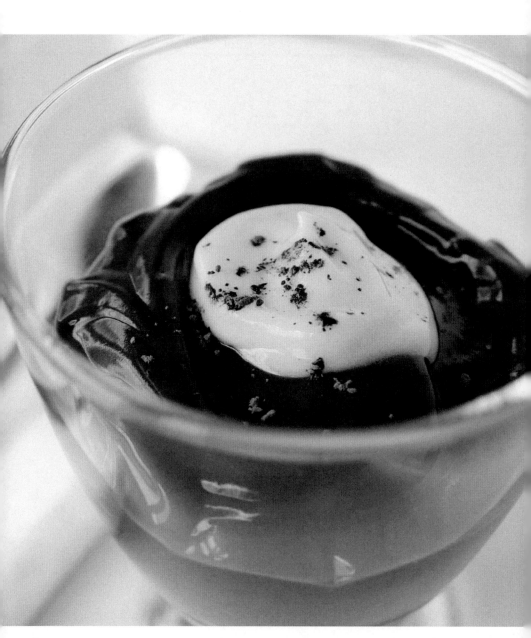

serves 6

3/4 cup coconut sugar

1/4 cup cornstarch

2 tablespoons cocoa powder

3 1/2 cups oat milk

4 ounces non-dairy semi-sweet chocolate, chopped

1 teaspoon vanilla extract

for hard sauce:

1/2 cup confectioners sugar

5 tablespoons non-dairy butter, softened

1 teaspoon vanilla

1/8 cup oat milk

1. In a mid-sized sauce pot, whisk together the sugar, cornstarch, and cocoa powder.

2. Gradually add the oat milk, whisking continuously to prevent lumping. Heat over medium heat, stirring continuously with a wooden spoon, and bring to a boil; boil for a couple of minutes.

3. Remove from heat and add chocolate. Stir until melted and add the vanilla.

4. Strain into a large bowl and separate into six individual cups.

5. Place in refrigerator until thoroughly chilled; about 1 to 2 hours.

directions for hard sauce:

6. Cream the butter; gradually add the confectioners sugar and beat until well blended; add oat milk and vanilla and blend smooth; chill until firm.

7. Scoop onto pudding before serving.

Tip: The hard sauce can be poured into a butter mold and sliced before serving for a more formal presentation.

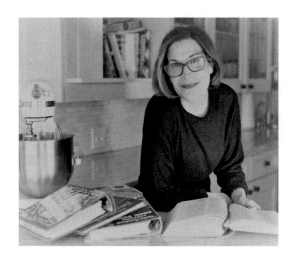

ABOUT THE AUTHOR

A Seattle-based culinary writer, **Laura Crotty** received her chef certification at the Institute for Culinary Education under the instruction of the late Annemarie Colbin, PhD, an early pioneer of the health-food movement. An ADDY Award recipient for her food journalism, her work has appeared in such outlets as Motherwell, the Huffington Post, and *Seattle Magazine*. Her interview subjects have included such luminaries as Chef Thomas Keller, the first and only American-born chef to hold multiple three-star ratings from the prestigious Michelin Guide; Alice Waters, owner of Chez Panisse and a pioneer of the farm to table movement in America; and Tom Douglas, restaurateur and multiple James Beard award recipient. This is her first book.

You can visit Laura @ lauracrotty.com.

Made in the USA
Monee, IL
30 January 2021